KARMA

KARMA

CHANGE YOUR LIFE

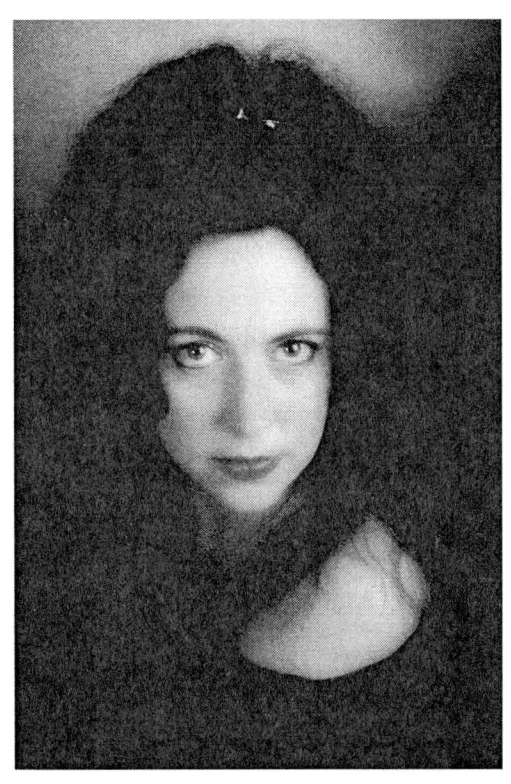

Rochelle Moore

Copyright © 2005 Rochelle Moore
All rights reserved.

ISBN : 1-4196-0939-4

To order additional copies, please contact us.
BookSurge, LLC
www.booksurge.com
1-866-308-6235
orders@booksurge.com

KARMA

To All Whom Down Through Time Have Kept These Secrets Of True Inner Life And Happiness For Others To Benefit

I would like to sincerely thank my very special family, my friends and everyone who has contributed to my experiences in this life which brought me to write this book.

A very special thanks to Richard, Shaun, Kyle, Tony Moore, Brid Moore, Orla, Niamh, Lily, Tom, Carmel, Katie, Emer and Dympna for their endless and all encompassing love. Also, thank you to RJ, Clarence, Gerry and Conor for their encouragement. Without these people I would not have had the many and varied experiences along my life's journey which are, to me, invaluable.

A special thank you to all at Fanstory who never gave up on me and spent their valued time polishing my work. To name but a few - Christine Jones, Duane Simolkie, Zen, Skye, Larry T, Hetty, Gayle, Louanne, Nescher Physcher, Lainee and Jock McFlurry. These people, like so many others in Fanstory are wonderful and insightful writers and poets, published and unpublished, whom deserve every success through their great Karmatic deeds.

Finally, thank you to all the countless men and women who, down through the ages, have perfected and preserved this wisdom. Thank you to all the animals and spiritual entities for your experiences and guidance.

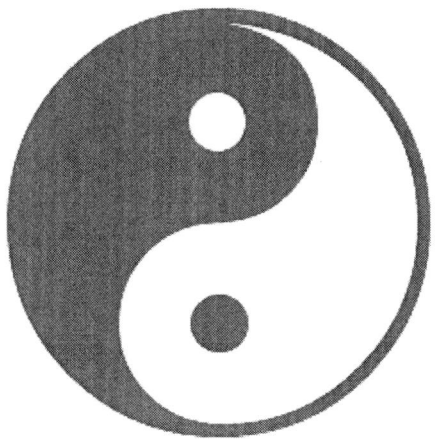

Rochelle Moore is a writer, a poet and above all, a dreamer. To date she has published poetry, short stories and is now concentrating on writing books and novels. Rochelle lives in Ireland - a writers paradise. She loves nature, animal rescue, Karma and horses. She is a very spiritual person who believes that there is good in everyone.

This book is written for those who feel that there is an alternative way in life and want to investigate different paths. Rochelle has written it as an introduction to Karma and has tried to keep it a light read. She has also dotted little poems here and there just for fun.

Her main ambition in life is to reach out to other peoples consciousness and if she even makes one person happy through her work she would feel that she accomplished her goal.

CONTENTS

This book shows you the way to a new and happier life

Awaken your true self
Inner Harmony
Feeling Safe
Meditation
Financial Flow
Letting Go
Look inside Yourself
Inner Power
Creative Expression
Environment
Mother Nature
Follow your true Path
Healing
Move Forward in Life
Peace of Mind
Resolve Problems
Guilt
Self-Reliance
Trusting Yourself
Tranquility
Honesty
Religions
Reincarnation

CHANGE YOUR LIFE

PROLOGUE

I have written this book as an introduction to the principals of Karma. The book is for people who want to be introduced to this very special way of life. I have divided the book into four parts as follows:

i. Basic structure of Karma
ii. Introduction to Karma
iii. Yin and Yang
iv. Karma in our daily lives

There is also a little poetry dotted here and there just for fun. Thank you for sharing my ways and may your Karma bring you health, wealth and success.

LOVE & LIGHT

PART 1

CAUSE & EFFECT

What goes around comes around. Goodness will be rewarded with goodness and evil with evil. Karma is the relationship between one's words, thoughts and actions. Karma advocates doing good works.

CAUSE MEANS REASON - EFFECT MEANS RESULT

INTRODUCTION

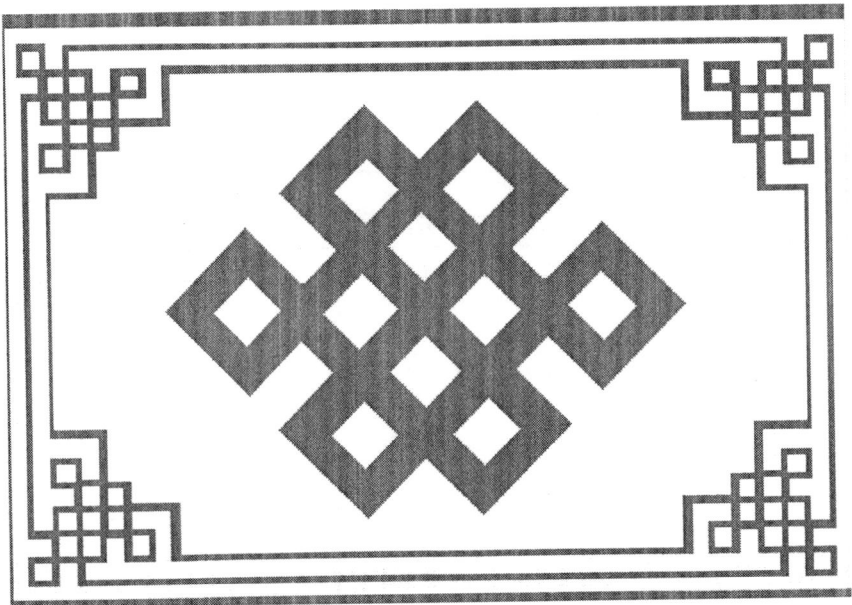

THE ENDLESS KNOT

If you accept your inner truth adhere to your path. The life force of the entire universe, is eternal. It gave birth to your soul, to all the planets and the solar system. This force is known by many names such as God, Jesus Christ, Angels, Avatars, Buddha, Islam, Krishna and many more. The point being that none of the above ways are wrong. These Deities are ever present. If you believe in one, all that is required from you is to follow your path with truth, faith and wisdom.

Thus, when you have no belief system or emit negative vibrations, you come up against a psychic energy barrier of positive vibrations - your own negativitity is bounced back. If you accept your inner voice of truth adhere to your path. Your own particular belief system is crucial for your well being. Wrongs should not have to be rationalised. You have your own free will and know right from wrong.

BUDDHA TAUGHT

"Do not think a small sin will not return in your future lives".

"Just as falling drops of water will fill a large container, the little sins that steadfast accumulate will completely overwhelm you".

"Do not think a small virtue will not return in your future lives".

"Just as falling drops of water will fill a large container, the little virtues that steadfast accumulate will completely overwhelm you."

THE ENDLESS KNOT

The endless knot symbolises the nature of reality where everything is interrelated and only exists as part of a web of Karma and its effect. It is endless and is also a symbol for long life.

This image signifies the interaction and interplay of opposing forces. This leads to their union and ultimately to harmony in the universe.

The knot represents a connection between our fates and our Karmatic destiny. This is one of the most favoured symbol of Tibetan Buddhism.

THE INFINITE WISDOM OF THE EARTH AND UNIVERSE

BUDDHIST KARMA

His holiness the Dalai Lama from 'Kindness, Clarity and Insight.

"Countless rebirths lie ahead, both good and bad. The effects of Karma (actions) are inevitable, and in previous lifetimes we have accumulated negative Karma which will inevitably have its fruition in this or future lives.

Just as someone witnessed by police in a criminal act will eventually be caught and punished, so we too must face the consequences of faulty actions we have committed in the past, there is no way to be at ease; those actions are irreversible; we all must eventually undergo their effects."

CONFUCIANISM

THE GOLDEN RULE OF CONFUCIANISM

(Extract from Tzu-Kung)

Tzu-Kung asked:-

"Is there one word which may serve as a rule of practice for all of one's life?".

Confucius answered:-

"Is not reciprocity such a word? What do you not want done to yourself, do not do to others".

THE BUDDHA

ANGUTTARA NIKAYA V-57

"I am the owner of my Karma.

I inherit my Karma
I am born with my Karma
I am related to my Karma
I live supported by my Karma

Whatever Karma I create, whether good or evil, that I shall inherit."

FOUR LAWS OF KARMA

RESULTS ARE SIMILAR TO CAUSE

Positive actions are defined as actions that have happiness as a result; negative actions are defined as actions that lead to suffering as a result

NO RESULTS WITHOUT CAUSE

As with the obvious facts behind Science, things do not just appear out of nothing.

ONCE AN ACTION IS DONE, THE RESULT IS NEVER LOST

Similar to above, things do not just disappear into nothing.

KARMA EXPANDS

Once we have an imprint of action in our minds, it tends to be habit forming. It then becomes normal.

FOUR LAWS OF PURIFICATION

POWER OF THE OBJECT

One should practice thinking of all beings one may have hurt. All sentient beings and the THREE JEWELS OF REFUGE, Buddha, Dharma and Shagha, generate compassion.

POWER OF REGRET

This should not be in the form of guilt which is a useless emotional torture. You should examine negative actions in the past and realise that you were very unwise.

POWER OF PROMISE

Promise not to repeat unwise negative actions and behaviour.

POWER OF PRACTICE

Any positive action with good motivation can be used as practice. Clear your field by purifying it from rocks and weeds. Plant anew.

MEDITATION

Sit or lie quietly and do not allow your impulses to have a mind of their own. Never be ruled by your impulses, as you have a life of your own.

Your impulses are not you - they are your thinking. By not reacting to them you come to understand their nature.

Meditation can alleviate destructive impulses. It can also enhance creative impulses. Nourish your mind, body and spirit by meditating for at least ten minutes daily. Your inner being will be awakened to a new experience and awareness.

NATURE

When we conspire against nature, disasters happen. If you maltreat the poor, the animals or Mother Nature, the result is natural imbalance.

When we abuse our abundant food supply by being greedy and consuming more than our share, the result is poverty and starvation.

If we are selfish for a long period of time, natural imbalance results in incidents of wars, epidemics, floods, famine and alterations in our weather and our earth.

BUDDHIST QUOTES

Do not speak - unless it improves on silence.

Your worst enemy cannot harm you as your own unguarded thoughts.

See the truth, and you will see me.

Love and compassion are necessary, not luxuries. Without them, humanity cannot survive.

It is under the greatest adversity that there exists the greatest potential for doing good, both for oneself and for others.

Anything that contradicts logic and experience should be abandoned.

The purpose of major religious traditions is not to construct big temples on the outside, but to create temples of goodness and compassion inside, in our hearts.

PART 2

KARMA

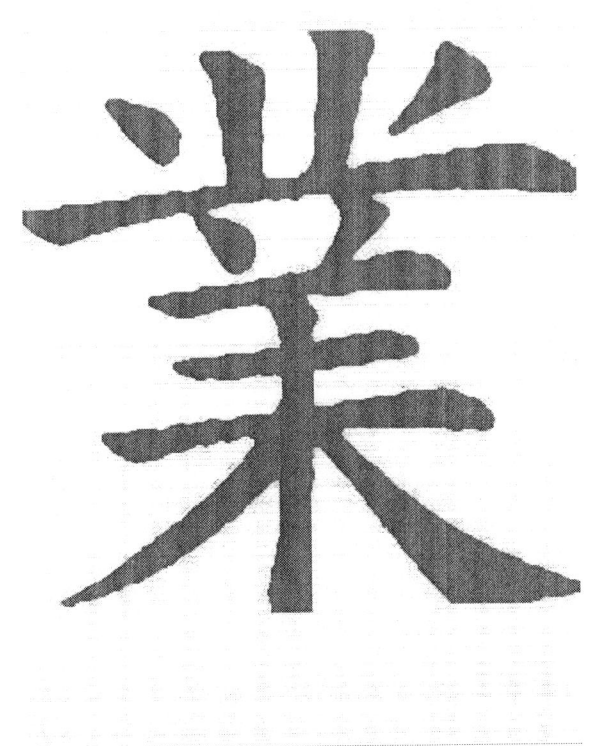

CHAPTERS 1 - 14

1. Cycles of Karma
2. Peace, Love & light
3. A Way of Life
4. Karmatic Tides
5. You are Perfect
6. Optimistic or Pessimistic?
7. Tranquility
8. Every breath you take is Precious
9. Pathways of Life
10. Positive Thinking
11. Negative Thinking
12. Ten Good Karma Rules
13. Ten Bad Karma Rules
14. Karma or Accident?

CYCLES OF KARMA

FOUNDATION

From birth to age 30 is the basis foundation laying period in Karma.

PRODUCTION

From age 30 to 50 is the production period within your Karmatic cycle.

REAPING YOUR REWARDS

From age 50 until death is the time to reap your Karmatic rewards. This is not a time for you to retire. It is the time for you to live your life to the fullest.

PEACE, LOVE & LIGHT

Keep your words and morals true.
All entities you mind.
Within your inner soul renew
the truth of all mankind.

Karma lies in all around,
no person, place nor thing.
To all, you see, it can be found
in nature's voice, will ring.

All beings of this universe
all creatures, humans, entities.
Your Karma lies for you to find
a path that sets you free.

(Copyright Rochelle Moore-2005)

A WAY OF LIFE

The word Karma literally means doing. Karma is more than a frame of mind, it is a way of life. This includes all physical and mental actions. We are a product of our own Karma. Karma advocates doing good works. This does not mean that you merely give away things that are of no value, nor giving alms to the poor and needy. Karma means that you continually sacrifice yourself. The result of good deeds not only benefits others, it benefits your life.

We are a product of our own Karma. Our actions and thoughts is our Karma. All energies that surround life emit vibrations, whether positive or negative. As we progress through life we gather these energies and they influence us in many ways.

For each action there is an equal and opposite reaction. Yin and Yang, male and female, good and evil. Karma can influence your lives in so many ways. Learning Karma is a way of changing your life.

KARMATIC TIDES

When you have the feeling that something is not right and you just don't know why, this is your deep inner super conscious voice trying to tell you that you are swimming against your Karmatic tide. Stop running on the spot and listen well to what your inner truth is trying to tell you. Just go with the flow and let your Karmatic tide redirect you. Be aware of your own inner feelings and hunches and follow the correct Karmatic path. Never doubt your inner truth.

An example of your super conscious looking after you is;

' Have you ever been driving along and suddenly think I don't remember driving for the past ten minutes?'.

Don't worry as you are completely safe. Your own super conscious mind is looking after you. This part of your mind would never allow anything to harm you and always looks out for your well being.

YOU ARE PERFECT

You are perfect in every way. All energies run in cycles. Always remember that you can tap into the universal power source through Karma. As Karma is timeless, eternal and all encompassing.

Mistakes: Are here to teach us lessons.

Accidents: Are here to redirect us back to our Karmatic destiny.

Disappointments: Are Karmatic tests.

It all balances out in the end. There is credit or deficit as all energies remain stable. All of your failures are temporary.

YOU ARE PERFECT

OPTIMISTIC OR PESSIMISTIC?

Every thought, every action, every feeling you have, affects your future Karma, for better or worse. An emotional reaction to shock can effect your health and your body's natural balance. Just as your body operates according to it's requirements and limitations, so does your Karmatic cycle and inner pattern.

Very bad news, such as divorce, a death, financial worry, can trigger depression. This can lead to a weakening of the immune system and further down the road, to a very serious illness. Just as an unexpected surprise or extreme excitement can result in lack of sleep, which in turn, can alter your well being.

Coping with major changes depends on whether you have an optimistic or a pessimistic view of life. Never ignore any major emotional changes. Look at every individual situation and learn from it. Karma is a great lesson teacher. Take every emotionally altering feeling and consider it a Karmatic challenge. Deal with it positively. Look for a resolution or solution. Be optimistic, not pessimistic.

CHANGE YOUR WORLD

TRANQUILITY

*Close your eyes and visualise
a place of love and peace.
Hear inside, a river's flow,
Let go, outside world, cease.
Prisms of vivid colours see.
Rainbows arching high.
Bright blue backdrop hovers calm,
a wondrous tranquil sky.*

*Let the outer world be gone.
Settle down and feel
the colours, peace, tranquillity.
Feel it, make it real.
Lay your body down to rest
upon the cool green grass.
Open up your inner eye,
in here, no time to pass.*

*The sound of water flowing.
The wondrous warming sun.
Settle now, your inner soul,
relax and be as one..
Watch the flitting butterfly
with enormous coloured wings.
Listen to the chorus
of the songbird as it sings.*

*With inner mind and spirit
Relax now, to your core.
Your body lies in perfect peace.
visit again, for more.
You open up your shiny eyes
and feel so fresh, anew.
A journey's end has come again.
Awaken tranquil through.*

(Copyright Rochelle Moore - 2005)

EVERY BREATH YOU TAKE IS PRECIOUS

Breathing in through your left nostril is your inner life.

Breathing out through your right nostril is your outer life.

Karma gives you perfect balance. Body, mind and Spirit. Find your balance and the true inner you.

ONLY THEN WILL TRUE INNER PEACE FOLLOW

PATHWAYS IN LIFE

*Measuring your path in life
your journey's, strife, be coy.
Begin a child, so innocent,
wondrous, so full of joy.*

*The system dictates your patterns.
Chisels, sculpts you with a knife.
Just who are they to sit and say,
what's wrong and what is right?*

*What makes a person normal?
Who's in charge to point the way?
Conform you must, or you'll go bust
socially and mentally, you'll pay.*

*So don't bother with what others think
Make your own reality.
Normal is as normal be
in this insecure society.*

*You find your pace, within your space.
Level out your soul and mind.
Forget the false harsh measures
muted out by humankind.*

*Choose your Karma wisely.
Be happy, live your life.
Once again, release the child,
forget the stress and strife.*

*Play, explore the inner you,
let the games begin.
Set your own reality
and you're the one who'll win.*

(Copyright Rochelle Moore - 2005)

POSITIVE THINKING

We receive what we send out whether positive or negative. Every thought is a self-fulfilling prophecy and becomes your reality. What we believe in we attract into our lives-whether positive or negative. If you really believe that you do not deserve something, you will not get it. If you believe that you are always ill, you will always be ill.

Thus, if you are positive in your thoughts you have the power to alter your life. Thinking positively will also benefit others as they are part of the universal mind. Like attracts like.

How many times have you heard of little miracles in your lifetime? Something or someone who as overcome all the odds stacked against them. Whether an illness, a change of fortune or a sudden cure. Positive energy and thoughts create your future.

THINK POSITIVE

NEGATIVE THINKING

Just as positive thinking can shape your future so can negative thinking. You have to clearly take responsibility or negate any negative thinking. If you have been emotionally hurt, try send love to the person who is responsible. If this love is rejected by them then their own energy will be returned to them.

If you have developed a pattern of negative thinking, you must change it immediately. If you think you are constantly ill, visualise wonderful health. Negative energy can drain your body and cause numerous illnesses. Media, movies, music, tell us subliminally what we are supposed to need. Your mind absorbs all this information and they become a very real part of your consciousness.

Start to change your negative thinking now and feel how quickly your life alters.

THINK POSITIVE

TEN GOOD RULES OF KARMA

1. Listen to Karmatic energy
2. Teach Karma to others
3. Rejoice in others good fortune
4. Service to others
5. Generosity
6. Reverence
7. Meditation
8. Restraint
9. Transference of Merit
10. Correction of our own errors

TEN BAD RULES OF KARMA

1. Killing another being or entity
2. Stealing
3. Sexual misconduct
4. Lying
5. Slander
6. Greed
7. Gossip
8. Anger
9. Cursing
10. Delusion

PLANNED OR ACCIDENTAL

Planning ahead in our lives makes for a better balance within this competitive world. We plan for most events such as, marriage, starting a family, we choose the type of work that is most beneficial for our survival, both financially and mentally. Today's pace of life is so fast we feel it very necessary to plan ahead even as far as our retirement. These plans make us feel more secure within our lives. They also make us feel that we are capable of dealing with any challenges that life throws our way.

Accidents? Do they exist? Or, is it the action that you select that causes accidents? Within Karma, nothing happens at random. Your thoughts, stresses and actions, influence all natural forces. You have created your present life by actions in your previous life. Karma means action. You reap what you sow. Most times accidents happen when you think you want or need something that in fact, would not be at all beneficial to you. Your Karmatic destiny will sometimes turn your thinking around and save you for whatever is your purpose in this life.

PART THREE

KARMA

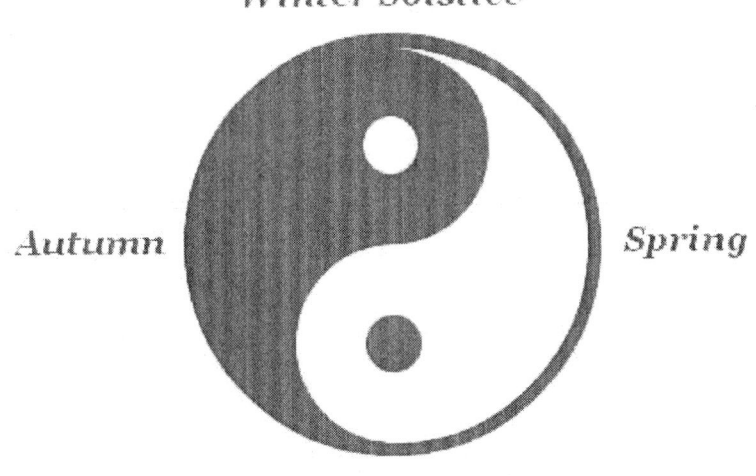

YIN & YANG

This symbol represents the ancient Chinese beliefs about how things work.

The outer circle represents everything. The black and white shapes within the circle represent the interaction of two energies - Yin and Yang. The Chinese believe that Yin (black) and Yang (white) cannot exist without each other. The two opposite energies within the one circle.

Yang: (white) is creative, upward, hot, strong and expanding.

Yin: (black) is passive, dark, cold, receptive and weak.

The Chinese determines four directions - *North, South, East and West*. By recording the Dipper's location in the sky and by watching the sun cast it's shadow from an eight foot pole, these seasonal changes were recorded thousands of years ago.

When the Dipper points East, it's Spring; when South, it's Summer; when West, it's Autumn; when North, it's Winter. The shortest shadow is at the Summer Solstice and the longer shadow is at the Winter Solstice.

The Chinese connected each line within a circle, Yin being part of the Summer Solstice and Yang's position to be part of the Winter Solstice and the above symbol emerged.

YIN & YANG

The dark colour area has less sunlight - Yin (moon). The light colour area has more sunlight- Yang (sun). Yin is like woman. Yang is like man. Neither can survive without the other. Yin could not give birth without Yang and vice-versa.

Yin begins at the Summer Solstice and Yang begins at the Winter Solstice. The two inner circles, which look like eyes, depicts that neither one could survive without the other. The outer circle contains it all together.

PERFECT HARMONY

YIN (WATER) - Forces of darkness, conservation, confusion and turmoil, shapes things and creates the senses.

YANG (FIRE) - Forces of light, destroys things, peace and serenity and disintegration.,

MIND, BODY & SPIRIT

Quotation by Qi Bo to the Yellow Emperor

"Yin and Yang are two energies that flow within your body.

When Yin is the stronger energy, you are cold and perspire with a chilling feeling. Your body becomes rebellious, your stomach can not digest food properly, which after a period can lead to grave illness, even death.

When Yang is the stronger energy, you are hot. Your pores close and you do not perspire. You become feverish, your stomach tightens, you become constipated, which after a period can also lead to grave illness, even death.

Only when you harmonise and adjust your body to these two principles of nature, will your body, soul and spirit, be in true balance".

MEDICAL THEORY

Quotation to the Yellow Emperor

"The principle of Yin & Yang is the Foundation of the entire universe. It is the root and source of life and of death. One must search for its origins".

Heaven was created by Yang, the force of light, earth was created by Yin, the force of darkness. If the female force is overwhelming, then there will be excessive cold. If the male force is overwhelming, then there will be excessive heat.

Exposure to either extremes of cold or heat, will cause disfunction in your body and the spirit will be injured.

Observe minute changes and treat them as if they are big and important. If treated, they will dissipate.

Harmony requires perfect balance".

PART FOUR

KARMA

CHAPTERS 13 - 36

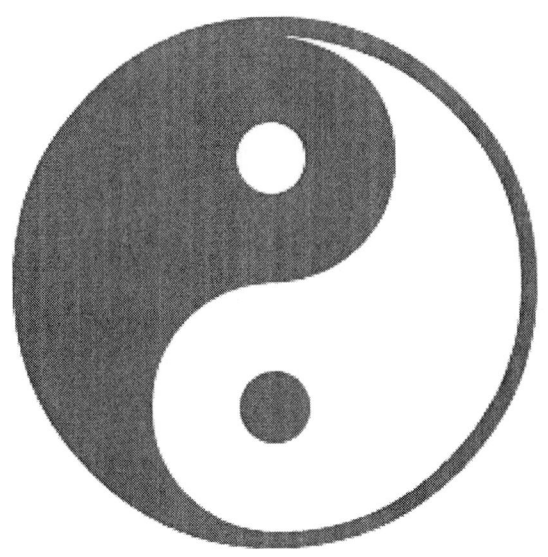

13. Types of Karma
14. Guidelines
15. Destiny
16. Gods
17. Jesus Christ
18. Buddha
19. Meditation

20. Prayer
21. Politics
22. Krishna
23. Religion
24. Reincarnation
25. Seven deadly Sins
26. Greed
27. Accomplish your Goals
28. Forgive and Forget
29. Compassion
30. Healing
31. Wisdom
32. Environment
33. Finance
34. Sowing and Reaping
35. Love
36. Health

TYPES OF KARMA

TWO TYPES OF KARMA

Karma has two kinds, this world and worldly.

OUTSIDE: Wisdom and detatchment.

WORLDLY: Good and evil.

You should strive to free yourself from all sorrow. Spend your time cultivating joy, happiness and wisdom to obtain great Karma. Always remember the rewards for good Karma and the retribution for evil Karma.

GUIDELINES

1. Follow the ten good Karma guidelines.
2. Regard other people, creatures and energies.
3. Sacrifice oneself for the universal good.
4. Perfect your own inner truth.
5. Cultivate the law of Karma within your life.
6. Release negative thoughts and energies.
7. Constantly strive to expand your good Karma.
8. Take care of nature and nurture all beings.
9. Meditate to awaken your inner being.
10. You are the owner of your own Karma.
11. Always remain optimistic.
12. Think positively and act positively.
13. Learn by your mistakes, resolve and solve.
14 Learn to be in complete harmony within.
15. You are perfect.

DESTINY

Watch your thoughts, for they become words. Watch your words, for they become actions.

Throughout all human life someone has always been our interpreter for any signs of destiny. Whether it be a mystic, a shaman, a doctor or any other type of pyschic. We all turn to some form of divination at some point in our lives. Can we therefore not assume that there must be something behind this?

Karma is the force beyond our minds as it determines true consciousness in itself. You can return to your destiny and practise Karma to enhance your life completely. You will get great results if you persevere.

LOVE & LIGHT

GOD'S

God's will is necessary and inevitable

Throughout all time, people have looked to their own particular God to assist within their life. We pray, we meditate, we go to pyschics, even philosophy has a place for these higher beings.

The secret of life is that it does not matter which of these beings you worship once you lead a full and committed spiritual life.

WHAT'S IN A NAME?

JESUS CHRIST

Jesus was a man who was wise and had the great ability to influence natural forces in our world. He learned to act carefully and utilise these powers for mankind. He could whip up a storm, part the sea and perform various 'miracles' by the power of thought.

Jesus died for the sins of humanity and we should repay him by trying to live good and honest lives. He thought that we, as the children of the devine Father in Heaven, or as children of the devine Father on earth, Jesus Christ, we have devine powers at our own disposal. When we sin against nature or mankind, we cause all kinds of dreadful events.

USE YOUR DIVINE POWER OF THOUGHT SKILFULLY

BUDDHA

KARMA AND REBIRTH

All living beings in the universe are alike. We are all subject to the same forces, energies and afflictions. Buddha taught that ignorance, attachment and aversion, whether a human trait, that of an animal or a being is not fated.

Buddha clearly states that Karma explains the different circumstances in which all living beings find themselves.

Karma is not predetermined. If you plant an Oak seed, it will grow and the result is an Oak tree.

AS YOU SOW YOU SHALL REAP

MEDITATION

"Quotes from Sogyal Rinpoche"

"It is extremely hard to rest undistracted in the nature of mind, even for a moment, let alone to self-liberate a single thought or emotion as it rises.

We often assume that simply because we understand something intellectually, - or think we do - that we have actually realised it. This is a great delusion.

It requires the maturity that only years of listening, contemplation, reflection and meditation, sustained practice can ripen".

BECOME YOUR OWN THERAPIST

PRAYER

Prayer is a very effective Karmatic act. You can send out your prayers to people around the world who are experiencing a catastrophy. No religion is required for this, just your own inner positive thinking.

If you are religious you can pray to your own God for troubled souls. You will help them a lot more than you think. Pray in a positive manner and ask for comfort for others. It is amazing what positive prayer can achieve.

BELIEVE IN PRAYER

POLITICS

Politics if not based on any Karmatic belief system. It is a man-made structure for the purpose of man. Politics can only be partially successful.

The answer to the world's problems is not political. It is usually politics that create the problems of the world in the first instance.

KARMA IS NOT POLITICAL

KRISHNA

Sir Krishna thought that in the spirit of Karma Yogi you should perform all acts that are necessary.

You should have a willingness to do your duty for no reward in this world.

ANCIENT BIBLES IN THE BHAGAVAD GITA

RELIGION

CORRECT THE PAST

DISCOVER THE PRESENT

CREATE THE FUTURE

In our past lives we have been many different spirits, races and part of many religions. We also have been both sexes.

Your religious beliefs are based on truth. If you have lived in so many other forms why have racism, religious wars or the battle of the sexes?

REINCARNATION

THE HOLY BIBLE

You are born to earth, live for a time in order to gain Karmatic experiences, pass away into spirit, dwell in spirit for a time, and are then reborn.

The Bible does have a few references to being left still, many have been omitted deliberately when the book was rewritten:-

JOHN THE BAPTIST - John - Chapter 1 - V24-25

The disciples enquired about John the Baptist

"If John was the Christ or Elijah, the profit returned?".

MATTHEW - Chapter 1 - V24-25

"Then Jesus said unto him, put up thy swords into it's place, for all that take the sword shall perish with the sword".

These chapters in the Bible relate to Karma, what goes around, coming back around in a future lifetime.

SEVEN DEADLY SINS

THE SINS - WHAT THEY SIN AGAINST

PRIDE - HUMANITY

GREED - GENEROSITY

ANGER - KINDNESS

ENVY - LOVE

GLUTTONY - FAITH

SLOTH - ZEAL

LUST - SELF CONTROL

ACCOMPLISH YOUR GOALS

As all thoughts end with a result believe that you can do anything. Never underestimate your own power and always be determined.

As you sow, so shall you reap. You get back exactly what you put out in life, and your thoughts are real things with energy.

Karma means doing. So you mentally and physically can do anything.

MEDITATE FOR SUCCESS

GREED

*To grip and grasp for gluttony
is a ghastly gruesome game.
Grief and graft for grubby goals,
for ghoulish ghostly gains.*

*Greatness is a Godsend,
Greed's glitter let's you down.
Glowing, gainly, gilted gifts,
you glorify a golden crown.*

*Get a grip and grap a grasp,
go generate some good.
Greed groups you in a
grotesque grave,
get out, and gather fast.*

*Growing gently, gone has greed.
Gratifying your soul.
Gleefully, growth sets you free
galvanising your new role.*

(Copyright Rochelle Moore - 2005)

FORGIVE AND FORGET

Whatever you give you will receive. In the world that we live in today, there are so many things that are so hard to forgive and forget. Karma does not forgive nor forget - it helps us and teaches us lessons.

As Karma is there to teach and not punish. We must learn a lesson. This is the reason why we are on earth. With this in mind you must try to forgive even the most dreadful of crimes. Try and send out your positive love to all of the victims. Even if you were a victim of crime.

Help guide me through the path of life. Show me what I still need to do. Help me to forgive and to forget.

COMPASSION

Never harm other humans, animals or energies which you cannot fathom. We are meant to look after each and every living thing on this earth. That is our duty.

Karma is compassionate. It always gives us hope. Although strict and unforgivable, you can still draw on Karma when you need it.

Ask God for a way of making amends for any of your wrongdoings. Find your solution and then make a resolution - then change your destiny.

HEALING

Karma can calm you, remove guilt, suffering, it can change your luck and it can also heal you.

Use your inner knowledge and meditate on the site that is ill. With your own words, gently concentrate on your ailment and improve it.

No matter what is wrong within your body you can use your wonderful source of power to heal.

The palms of your hands are transmitters. Place your hands over the area and transmit love, understanding, energy and inner light - heal yourself.

WISDOM

Some say that you are born with it,
a gift, not to be wasted.
Others say, it must be earned,
savoured well and tasted.

Wisdom can't be earned by fools,
no matter how they try.
I believe that wisdom's sight
comes from your inner eye.

Born with a gift to treasure,
To build, nourish and grow.
Once a weed always a weed
that's Mother Nature's blow.

T'is not confined to humankind
this treasure reaches all.
The secret of inner wisdom
a sacred and wondrous call.

Remember now your duty
if wisdom you've been granted.
Use it well, don't waste nor quell
share with man and animal.
This ancient inner knowledge tell
to all who need a warning bell.

(Copyright Rochelle Moore - 2005)

ENVIRONMENT

Your environment and your surroundings should be treated as Heaven on earth. Feelings and tolerance are essential within your life.

No matter where you live, what colour, race or religious belief system that you hold dear, never defy your environment.

CHERISH IT

FINANCE

Karma states that what you give out will be returned. This applies to every area of your life, including finance.

So, if you are having financial problems give something away. Give to another more needy than you. It matters little the amount.

GIVE AND YOU SHALL RECEIVE

SOWING AND REAPING

You get back exactly what you put out. As you sow, you shall reap. As you reap, you shall sow.

Karma teaches us that we must learn from all of our actions whether mental or physical.

SOW WISELY AND YOU SHALL REAP ABUNDANTLY

LOVE

You cannot possess love if you submit it to rigid structure. If you love someone you must allow complete freedom. Through this freedom, if love is then offered back to you, it is real.

What you give out you will receive back. Give your love unconditionally and you will receive love unconditionally.

LET YOUR LOVE BE FREE

HEALTH

We are all responsible for our own being. It is our Karmatic duty to look after our body, mind and spirit.

Meditate, be positive, treat your body like a temple.

BECOME YOUR OWN HEALER

APPENDIX

Now that you have read how to change your life through Karma, how to overcome fear, failure, guilt and suffering put it to good use. Bathe in the peace, tranquillity and growth of your Karma. There is nothing to fear but fear itself. Any failures are temporary and are a Karmatic lesson. Learn from your failures.

If you feel guilty about something, it means that you have a conscience. That's good! If you are ill, heal yourself. If others are suffering, help them. Observe your mind, body and spirit and listen to your inner truth.

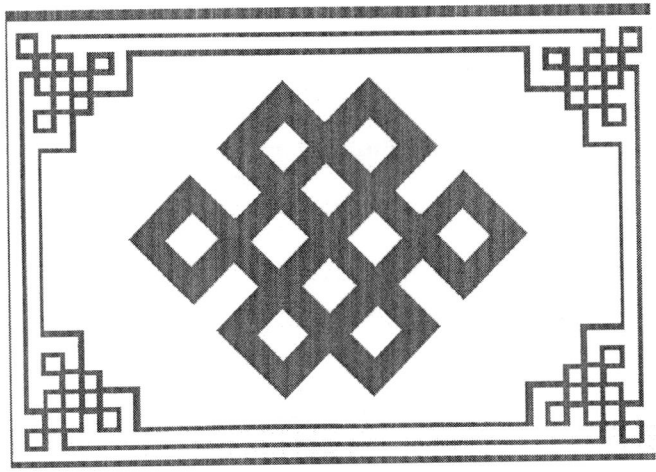

MAY YOUR DESTINY FULFILL YOU. PEACE, LOVE & LIGHT.

EPILOGUE

I hope that this book can help you on your journey through this life. Karma can help your to clarify decisions through understanding, remove any habits or mental blocks that you have created, make your journey a happy and harmonious one and remove negativity from your life completely.

This book will enhance your entire being. With a bit of practice you will come to understand your deepest fears, emotional imbalances and through your own interpretation, change your life for good.

If you introduce Karma into your lives you will soon notice minor to major changes in your day-to-day life. You will find happiness, harmony, healing and make the world a better place. Karma is real and is very powerful. It will put your mind in a place that is tranquil and will clarify global worldly matters which are created by man.

It is very important to note that you can alter your future through your thoughts. The habits that have brought you to this book today can be altered and by selecting to read this book means that you are currently searching for a new and better way of life. No longer will you self-sabotage your joy and you can now move forward and change your lifestyle and thought patterns and focus on your future.

I hope that you have enjoyed this book and if you would like any further information, please contact:

KASHMIR INTERNTIONAL

ROCKBROOK HOUSE
BROOKFIELD TERRACE
BLACKROCK
CO DUBLIN
IRELAND.

FAX: 00 353 1 2883293

Or, contact Rochelle via email @: Rochelle.Moore@homail.com

PEACE, LOVE & LIGHT